Welcome to

I0792314

Fast Food in America
"The Health Effects, Cultural Impacts, and Future of Convenience Eating"

By: Clarence E. Riley

The story of fast food is one of innovation, adaptation, and consequences—a narrative that mirrors the challenges and opportunities of contemporary society!

Fast Food in America
"The Health Effects, Cultural Impacts, and Future of Convenience Eating"

Table of Contents

Fast Food in America
"The Health Effects, Cultural Impacts, and Future of Convenience Eating"

Introduction

Fast food has become a defining feature of modern American life, influencing not only what we eat but also how we live. Its rise is deeply intertwined with the nation's history, from industrialization and urbanization to changes in family dynamics and work habits. What began as a simple solution to a need for quick, affordable meals has grown into a multibillion-dollar industry that shapes our health, culture, and even our future.

The origins of fast food can be traced back to the early 20th century, during a time when the United States was rapidly industrializing. As cities expanded and more Americans moved into urban areas, the demand for convenient, ready-to-eat meals grew. Fast food met this need by offering quick service and consistent products. The model thrived on efficiency, simplicity, and affordability, aligning perfectly with the fast-paced lives of workers and families. By the mid-20th century, fast food was firmly embedded in American culture, reflecting a society increasingly focused on convenience and time management.

Over the decades, fast food has had a profound impact on health. While it initially presented itself as a practical dining solution, its emphasis on affordability and flavor often came at the expense of nutritional value. Meal's rich in fats, sugars, and sodium became staples, contributing to widespread health challenges. The correlation between fast food consumption and conditions such as obesity, heart disease, and diabetes has been the subject of extensive research, highlighting the long-term consequences of a diet dominated by convenience foods.

Fast Food in America
"The Health Effects, Cultural Impacts, and Future of Convenience Eating"

Culturally, fast food has played a pivotal role in shaping American identity. It embodies the ideals of efficiency and accessibility, offering a taste of modernity and progress. At the same time, it has influenced social dynamics, from the way families gather around meals to how communities interact with food. Fast food establishments became gathering places, symbols of affordability, and a reflection of the nation's evolving lifestyle.

Looking to the future, the role of fast food continues to evolve in response to changing societal priorities. The rise of health-conscious movements, concerns about environmental sustainability, and technological advancements are reshaping the industry. Alternatives to traditional fast food are gaining popularity, offering options that balance convenience with health and ecological responsibility.

This book delves into the intricate relationship between fast food and American life, exploring its health effects, cultural impacts, and potential future. By understanding the past and present of fast food, we can better navigate its role in our lives and make informed choices for the years ahead. This journey is not only about what we eat but also about the values we uphold and the future we envision.

Fast Food in America
"The Health Effects, Cultural Impacts, and Future of Convenience Eating"

Chapter 1

The Evolution of Fast Food in America

☐ Origins of fast food and its rise in popularity.

☐ Cultural shifts that made fast food a staple of American dining.

☐ How industrialization and urbanization set the stage for its success.

Fast food has become an integral part of American culture, representing a lifestyle that values speed, efficiency, and convenience. Its story is deeply rooted in the nation's history, shaped by social, economic, and technological changes that transformed how people eat and live. From its humble beginnings to becoming a cornerstone of modern dining, fast food's evolution reflects broader societal trends and cultural shifts that have defined the American experience.

Origins of Fast Food and Its Rise in Popularity

The origins of fast food in America can be traced back to the late 19th and early 20th centuries, a period of immense change marked by rapid industrialization and urbanization. As cities expanded, so did the need for quick, affordable meals for workers who had little time to prepare food at home. Early forms of fast food appeared in urban areas, where vendors sold simple, ready-to-eat items that catered to busy lifestyles. These offerings were inexpensive and accessible, appealing to a growing population of urban dwellers.

Fast Food in America
"The Health Effects, Cultural Impacts, and Future of Convenience Eating"

By the early 20th century, the concept of fast food began to solidify with the introduction of standardized menus and assembly-line food preparation techniques. These innovations made it possible to produce meals quickly and consistently, meeting the needs of an increasingly mobile and time-conscious society. As transportation systems improved, fast food establishments began to appear along major roadways, catering to travelers and commuters. This marked the beginning of a national expansion that would redefine American dining.

During the mid-20th century, fast food became synonymous with modernization and progress. Advances in food preservation, packaging, and distribution allowed fast food to reach new markets, from suburban neighborhoods to rural communities. The rise of car culture in the United States further propelled the industry, as drive-in and drive-through establishments catered to a society on the move. By the 1950s and 1960s, fast food had become a symbol of American ingenuity and convenience, embraced by people from all walks of life.

Cultural Shifts That Made Fast Food a Staple of American Dining

The rise of fast food in America coincided with significant cultural shifts that reshaped the nation's dining habits. One of the most influential factors was the changing structure of the American family. As more women entered the workforce during and after World War II, traditional home-cooked meals became less feasible for many households. Fast food provided a practical alternative, offering meals that required little preparation time and fit into busy schedules.

The post-war economic boom also played a key role in fast food's ascent. Rising incomes and the growth of suburban living

Fast Food in America
"The Health Effects, Cultural Impacts, and Future of Convenience Eating"

created a demand for dining options that were affordable, convenient, and accessible. Fast food establishments quickly adapted to this new landscape, offering menu items that appealed to a broad audience and locations that were easy to reach. The standardization of recipes and branding further solidified fast food's place in the American diet, creating a sense of familiarity and reliability for consumers.

Cultural trends also contributed to the popularity of fast food. The mid-20th century saw the emergence of a youth-oriented culture that valued individuality and leisure. Fast food establishments became gathering places for young people, offering an informal and affordable space to socialize. This cultural association with youth and modernity helped fast food gain a foothold in American society, making it a preferred choice for generations of diners.

How Industrialization and Urbanization Set the Stage for Its Success

The success of fast food in America is deeply tied to the nation's industrial and urban development. The industrial revolution brought about significant changes in food production, transportation, and labor, creating the conditions necessary for fast food to thrive. Mass production techniques, such as assembly lines, revolutionized the way food was prepared and served, enabling fast food establishments to produce meals quickly and efficiently. This approach not only reduced costs but also ensured consistency, which became a hallmark of the industry.

Urbanization further fueled the demand for fast food. As cities grew, so did the number of people who needed convenient dining options. The dense population of urban areas provided a

Fast Food in America
"The Health Effects, Cultural Impacts, and Future of Convenience Eating"

ready market for fast food establishments, which could serve large numbers of customers in a short amount of time. The rise of public transportation and automobiles also made it easier for people to access fast food, contributing to its widespread appeal.

Technological advancements played a crucial role in the evolution of fast food. Innovations in refrigeration, food processing, and packaging extended the shelf life of ingredients and allowed for centralized production and distribution. These developments enabled fast food companies to streamline operations and expand their reach, bringing their offerings to a national audience. The introduction of modern kitchen equipment, such as fryers and grills, further enhanced the speed and efficiency of food preparation.

Fast food's success was also bolstered by changes in agricultural practices. The shift towards industrial farming and the development of high-yield crops ensured a steady supply of ingredients at low costs. These agricultural advancements supported the mass production of fast food, making it an affordable option for consumers and a profitable venture for businesses.

The Social and Economic Impacts of Early Fast Food

As fast food gained popularity, it began to influence broader social and economic trends in America. The industry created new opportunities for employment, particularly for young and unskilled workers. Fast food establishments became a significant source of jobs, offering entry-level positions that required minimal training. This accessibility made fast food an important stepping stone for many individuals entering the workforce.

Fast Food in America
"The Health Effects, Cultural Impacts, and Future of Convenience Eating"

Economically, fast food contributed to the growth of related industries, including agriculture, transportation, and food processing. The demand for ingredients, packaging materials, and distribution networks created a ripple effect that supported economic development across multiple sectors. Fast food also played a role in shaping consumer behavior, introducing concepts such as value meals, combo deals, and limited-time offers that influenced purchasing patterns.

Socially, the rise of fast food reflected changing attitudes towards dining and leisure. The convenience and affordability of fast food made it a popular choice for families, workers, and travelers, offering a solution to the challenges of modern life. Fast food establishments became cultural landmarks, representing a new era of dining that prioritized speed and efficiency over tradition.

A Cultural Phenomenon in the Making

By the latter half of the 20th century, fast food had become more than just a dining option; it was a cultural phenomenon. Its influence extended beyond the plate, shaping advertising, entertainment, and even fashion. The bright colors, catchy slogans, and iconic imagery associated with fast food became symbols of American culture, recognized and emulated around the world.

At its core, the evolution of fast food in America is a story of adaptation and innovation. It reflects the nation's ability to respond to changing needs and priorities, using technology and creativity to redefine the way people eat. While fast food has its critics, its impact on American life is undeniable, offering insights into the complexities of modern society and the choices we make as consumers.

Fast Food in America
"The Health Effects, Cultural Impacts, and Future of Convenience Eating"

Looking Ahead

Understanding the origins and evolution of fast food provides a foundation for exploring its broader implications. As this book continues, we will examine the health effects, cultural impacts, and future possibilities of convenience eating. By reflecting on the past, we can gain a deeper appreciation for the role fast food plays in our lives and consider how it might evolve in the years to come. This journey is not only about food but also about the values and priorities that define us as individuals and as a society.

Fast Food in America
"The Health Effects, Cultural Impacts, and Future of Convenience Eating"

Chapter 2

The Nutritional Reality of Fast Food

- ☐ Common ingredients and nutritional profiles of fast food.

- ☐ The role of processed foods, additives, and high-calorie meals.

- ☐ Examination of portion sizes and their implications for health.

Fast food is a defining feature of modern dietary habits, offering convenience and affordability. However, its nutritional reality is a topic of growing concern. By examining the ingredients, nutritional profiles, and implications of portion sizes, we can better understand how fast-food impacts health and why it continues to be a focal point of nutritional discourse.

Common Ingredients and Nutritional Profiles of Fast Food

Fast food relies heavily on a set of staple ingredients chosen for their cost-effectiveness, shelf stability, and taste appeal. These ingredients often include refined carbohydrates, fats, sodium, and sugars. The emphasis on flavor and texture often comes at the expense of nutrient density, leaving many fast-food options high in calories but low in essential vitamins and minerals.

Fast Food in America
"The Health Effects, Cultural Impacts, and Future of Convenience Eating"

One of the defining characteristics of fast food is its reliance on refined carbohydrates. These include white bread buns, pasta, and other starches that have been stripped of their natural fiber and nutrients. Refined carbohydrates are quickly digested, leading to rapid spikes in blood sugar and insulin levels. This can contribute to energy crashes and long-term health issues like type 2 diabetes.

Fats play a significant role in the flavor profile of fast food. Often derived from hydrogenated oils, these fats include trans fats and saturated fats. Although trans fats are being phased out due to their known health risks, many fast-food items remain high in saturated fats, which are linked to increased levels of LDL cholesterol and heart disease.

Sodium is another ubiquitous ingredient in fast food, used both as a preservative and a flavor enhancer. While sodium is an essential mineral, excessive intake can lead to high blood pressure, kidney strain, and other cardiovascular issues. The average fast-food meal often contains more than half the recommended daily intake of sodium, making moderation challenging for frequent consumers.

Sugars and sweeteners are heavily utilized in fast food beverages, desserts, and even savory dishes. High-fructose corn syrup and other added sugars contribute to calorie overload without providing satiety, often encouraging overconsumption.

Fast Food in America
"The Health Effects, Cultural Impacts, and Future of Convenience Eating"

The Role of Processed Foods, Additives, and High-Calorie Meals

Fast food is synonymous with processed food, which is designed for rapid preparation and long shelf life. Processing methods often involve the addition of preservatives, artificial flavors, and stabilizers, all of which serve to enhance the food's appeal and longevity. However, these additives can have unintended consequences for health.

Preservatives such as nitrates and nitrites, commonly found in processed meats, have been associated with potential health risks when consumed in excess. Artificial flavors and colors, while generally deemed safe for consumption, raise concerns about their cumulative effects over time, especially in populations with high fast-food consumption.

The caloric density of fast-food meals is another point of concern. Many fast food options pack a significant number of calories into small portions, often due to the combination of fats and sugars. High-calorie meals contribute to the growing issue of obesity, particularly when consumed regularly without offsetting physical activity. The energy imbalance created by these meals exacerbates the risk of chronic conditions such as cardiovascular disease and metabolic syndrome.

Fast Food in America
"The Health Effects, Cultural Impacts, and Future of Convenience Eating"

Examination of Portion Sizes and Their Implications for Health

Portion sizes in fast food establishments have increased significantly over the decades, paralleling the rise in obesity rates. Larger portions are marketed as better value for money, encouraging consumers to eat more than they need. This "supersizing" phenomenon has normalized excessive caloric intake, contributing to a culture of overconsumption.

For example, what was once considered a standard serving size for a beverage or side dish is now often marketed as a "small" option. The availability of larger sizes creates a psychological anchor, making smaller portions seem insufficient. Additionally, many fast-food meals bundle high-calorie sides and sugary drinks into combos, further increasing overall caloric intake.

The impact of portion sizes on health is profound. Consuming oversized portions regularly can lead to gradual weight gain, even in individuals who are otherwise active. Excess calorie intake from these meals often goes unnoticed, as fast food is engineered to be highly palatable and easy to consume quickly. This can hinder the body's natural hunger and fullness signals, leading to overeating.

Beyond caloric intake, the imbalance of macronutrients in fast food portion sizes also affects health. Meals disproportionately high in fats and carbohydrates can disrupt metabolic processes, leading to insulin resistance and fat accumulation. The lack of fiber and protein—nutrients that promote satiety—further exacerbates the cycle of overeating and poor nutrition.

The Psychological and Societal Factors Behind Fast Food Consumption

Understanding the nutritional reality of fast food requires consideration of the psychological and societal factors that drive its consumption. Fast food is marketed as a convenient, affordable option for individuals and families. Its accessibility makes it an easy choice, particularly for those with limited time or financial resources.

The sensory appeal of fast food also plays a role. Its flavors, textures, and presentation are carefully designed to trigger pleasure centers in the brain, creating a rewarding eating experience. This can lead to habitual consumption, as individuals seek the convenience and satisfaction that fast food provides.

On a societal level, the ubiquity of fast-food outlets and advertising reinforces its role as a staple of modern life. This normalization can make it challenging to prioritize healthier eating habits, particularly in environments where fast food is the most convenient or affordable option.

The Path Forward

The nutritional reality of fast food underscores the need for greater awareness and education about its effects on health. While fast food offers undeniable convenience, its

Fast Food in America
"The Health Effects, Cultural Impacts, and Future of Convenience Eating"

long-term impact on health is a growing concern. Addressing these issues requires a multi-faceted approach that includes individual choices, public health initiatives, and industry reform.

For individuals, moderation and informed decision-making can help mitigate the risks associated with fast food consumption. Choosing smaller portions, prioritizing options with lower sodium and added sugars, and balancing fast food meals with nutrient-dense home-cooked meals are practical steps.

Public health campaigns can also play a role in raising awareness about the nutritional pitfalls of fast food. By promoting education about portion sizes, caloric intake, and the importance of balanced diets, these initiatives can empower consumers to make healthier choices.

Finally, the fast-food industry itself has a role to play in improving nutritional standards. Offering smaller portion sizes, reducing the use of harmful additives, and providing transparency about nutritional content can help consumers make more informed decisions. Some progress has been made in these areas, but there is still significant room for improvement.

Conclusion

The nutritional reality of fast food highlights the complexities of balancing convenience with health. While fast food fulfills a need for quick, affordable meals, its reliance on high-calorie, low-nutrient ingredients poses

Fast Food in America
"The Health Effects, Cultural Impacts, and Future of Convenience Eating"

challenges for long-term health. By understanding these dynamics and taking proactive steps, both individuals and society can work toward a healthier relationship with fast food.

Fast Food in America
"The Health Effects, Cultural Impacts, and Future of Convenience Eating"

Chapter 3

Fast Food and Obesity

- ☐ Connections between fast food consumption and obesity rates.

- ☐ How calorie-dense, nutrient-poor meals contribute to weight gain.

- ☐ Discussion of societal and individual consequences of obesity.

The modern obesity epidemic has become one of the most pressing public health challenges, and its connection to fast food consumption has been the subject of intense scrutiny. Obesity, characterized by an excess of body fat that poses risks to health, is influenced by a complex interplay of factors, including diet, lifestyle, genetics, and environment. Fast food—known for its calorie-dense, nutrient-poor offerings—plays a significant role in this multifaceted issue. Understanding the links between fast food consumption and obesity requires an examination of dietary habits, the nutritional composition of fast food, and the broader societal implications.

The Caloric Density of Fast Food

Fast food is often designed to be hyper-palatable, combining high levels of sugar, fat, and salt to enhance taste and encourage repeat consumption. These foods are typically calorie-dense, meaning they provide a high number of calories relative to their weight. This caloric density is a significant contributor to excessive calorie intake, especially when individuals consume large portions or pair main dishes with calorie-heavy sides and beverages.

The energy imbalance—consuming more calories than are expended through physical activity and basal metabolic processes—is a primary driver of weight gain. Fast food's convenient and inexpensive nature makes it accessible to a broad population, but its frequent consumption can lead to sustained caloric surpluses, resulting in gradual but consistent weight gain over time.

Nutrient-Poor Meals and Satiety

Fast food meals are often low in essential nutrients like fiber, vitamins, and minerals. Fiber, for example, plays a crucial role in promoting satiety and regulating appetite. A lack of fiber in fast food meals means that individuals may feel less satisfied after eating, which can lead to increased calorie consumption later in the day. Additionally, the high levels of refined carbohydrates and added sugars in many fast-food items can cause rapid spikes and subsequent drops in blood sugar levels, further driving hunger and overeating.

Moreover, the absence of nutrient diversity in fast food contributes to its poor overall dietary quality. While it provides energy in the form of calories, it often fails to deliver the necessary nutrients required for optimal health. This imbalance can contribute to the development of obesity and associated health conditions such as type 2 diabetes, cardiovascular disease, and metabolic syndrome.

Fast Food in America
"The Health Effects, Cultural Impacts, and Future of Convenience Eating"

Portion Sizes and Their Implications

Portion sizes in fast food establishments have increased dramatically over the decades. This phenomenon, often referred to as "portion distortion," has normalized larger serving sizes, making it difficult for individuals to recognize appropriate portions. Studies have shown that larger portions encourage people to eat more, regardless of their actual hunger levels. This behavioral tendency, combined with fast food's low cost and high palatability, amplifies the risk of overeating.

Large portion sizes also blur the perception of what constitutes a single meal. For instance, what was once considered an indulgence is now marketed as a standard meal, further ingraining excessive calorie consumption into dietary habits. The affordability of upsized meals and bundled deals exacerbates this issue, making it economically appealing for individuals to consume larger quantities of food.

Fast Food and Childhood Obesity

Children and adolescents are particularly vulnerable to the effects of fast-food consumption. The prevalence of childhood obesity has risen in parallel with the expansion of fast-food availability. Factors such as aggressive marketing strategies targeting young audiences, the incorporation of toys and other incentives with meals, and the proximity of fast-food outlets to schools contribute to the high rates of fast food consumption among youth.

The dietary patterns established during childhood often persist into adulthood, meaning that early exposure to high-calorie, nutrient-poor fast food can set the stage for lifelong health challenges. Obese children are more likely to become obese

Fast Food in America
"The Health Effects, Cultural Impacts, and Future of Convenience Eating"

adults, facing an elevated risk of chronic diseases and reduced quality of life.

Societal Consequences of Obesity

The societal impact of obesity is profound, affecting not only individuals but also families, communities, and healthcare systems. Obesity-related health conditions, such as hypertension, diabetes, and heart disease, place a significant burden on public health resources. The economic costs associated with treating these conditions, along with the loss of productivity due to obesity-related disabilities, are substantial.

Social stigma and discrimination against individuals with obesity further compound the problem. Weight bias can affect employment opportunities, mental health, and access to quality healthcare. This stigma often creates a cycle of poor self-esteem and unhealthy behaviors, perpetuating the challenge of managing weight effectively.

Individual Consequences of Obesity

For individuals, obesity can lead to a wide range of physical, emotional, and psychological challenges. Physically, the excess weight increases the strain on joints and the cardiovascular system, leading to a higher risk of osteoarthritis, sleep apnea, and other health issues. Obesity is also closely linked to certain types of cancer, reproductive issues, and reduced life expectancy.

Emotionally, individuals with obesity may experience anxiety, depression, and low self-esteem. These mental health challenges are often exacerbated by societal stigma and personal struggles with weight management. Psychological

Fast Food in America
"The Health Effects, Cultural Impacts, and Future of Convenience Eating"

stress can also contribute to disordered eating patterns, creating a feedback loop that hinders efforts to adopt healthier lifestyles.

Urbanization and Fast-Food Access

The rise of urbanization has facilitated the proliferation of fast-food outlets, particularly in densely populated areas. Urban environments often present barriers to accessing fresh, healthy foods, leading to a reliance on convenient options like fast food. In many communities, fast food outlets are more accessible than grocery stores or markets offering fresh produce. This phenomenon, often described as living in a "food desert," disproportionately affects low-income populations, exacerbating health disparities and contributing to higher obesity rates in these communities.

The Role of Education and Awareness

While fast food consumption is a significant factor in the obesity epidemic, education and awareness play a crucial role in mitigating its impact. Public health campaigns and nutrition education programs can empower individuals to make informed dietary choices, understand portion sizes, and recognize the importance of balanced meals. Labeling initiatives, such as displaying calorie counts and nutritional information, aim to increase transparency and help consumers make healthier decisions when dining out.

However, education alone is not sufficient to address the systemic factors that contribute to obesity. Broader efforts to improve access to healthy foods, regulate advertising practices, and promote active lifestyles are essential components of a comprehensive strategy to combat obesity.

Fast Food in America
"The Health Effects, Cultural Impacts, and Future of Convenience Eating"

Future Directions and Solutions

Addressing the link between fast food and obesity requires a multifaceted approach. Policymakers, healthcare providers, educators, and community leaders must work together to create environments that support healthy eating habits. Potential strategies include implementing taxes on sugary beverages, subsidizing fruits and vegetables, and encouraging the development of urban agriculture initiatives.

On an individual level, fostering a culture of mindful eating and encouraging home-cooked meals can help reduce reliance on fast food. Innovations in the food industry, such as the development of healthier fast-food options and plant-based alternatives, also hold promise for mitigating the health impacts of fast-food consumption.

Conclusion

The connection between fast food and obesity highlights the broader challenges of maintaining a healthy diet in a modern, convenience-driven society. While fast food offers undeniable advantages in terms of accessibility and affordability, its role in promoting calorie-dense, nutrient-poor eating habits cannot be overlooked. Addressing this issue requires a collective effort to balance the convenience of fast food with the imperative of promoting public health. By understanding the factors that contribute to obesity and implementing targeted solutions, society can work toward a healthier future while preserving the benefits of convenience eating.

Fast Food in America
"The Health Effects, Cultural Impacts, and Future of Convenience Eating"

Chapter 4

Chronic Health Issues Linked to Fast Food

☐ Links to conditions such as diabetes, heart disease, and hypertension.

☐ The impact of excessive sodium, sugars, and unhealthy fats.

☐ Long-term effects of frequent consumption on physical health.

Fast food has long been associated with various chronic health conditions that affect millions of individuals worldwide. Its convenience and affordability often come at the expense of nutritional quality, leading to significant health implications over time. This chapter explores the connections between fast food consumption and chronic illnesses such as diabetes, heart disease, and hypertension, while also examining the roles of excessive sodium, sugars, and unhealthy fats in these conditions. Finally, it addresses the long-term effects of frequent fast-food consumption on physical health.

Links to Chronic Conditions

One of the most significant health concerns associated with fast food consumption is the rise in type 2 diabetes. The high levels of refined carbohydrates and added sugars commonly found in fast food items can cause sharp spikes in blood sugar levels, leading to insulin resistance over time. Insulin resistance is a hallmark of type 2 diabetes, a condition that requires lifelong

Fast Food in America
"The Health Effects, Cultural Impacts, and Future of Convenience Eating"

management and can result in severe complications such as nerve damage, kidney failure, and vision loss.

Heart disease is another prevalent health issue linked to fast food. Meal's rich in trans fats, saturated fats, and cholesterol can contribute to the buildup of plaque in the arteries, a condition known as atherosclerosis. This narrowing of the arteries reduces blood flow, increasing the risk of heart attacks and strokes. Additionally, the excessive sodium content in fast food items can raise blood pressure, a leading cause of hypertension and a significant risk factor for cardiovascular diseases.

Hypertension, or high blood pressure, is exacerbated by the excessive sodium levels in fast food. Many fast-food meals contain more than the recommended daily intake of sodium in a single serving. This excessive sodium can cause water retention, placing extra strain on blood vessels and the heart. Over time, chronic high blood pressure can lead to organ damage, including heart failure and kidney disease.

The Role of Sodium, Sugars, and Unhealthy Fats

Fast food is often laden with ingredients that contribute to its palatability and extended shelf life but also have detrimental effects on health. Sodium, for example, is used extensively as a preservative and flavor enhancer. While the body needs a certain amount of sodium to function, excessive intake disrupts the delicate balance of electrolytes and fluids, leading to hypertension and an increased risk of stroke.

Sugars are another major component of fast food, particularly in beverages, desserts, and condiments. The overconsumption of added sugars can lead to weight gain, increased fat accumulation in the liver, and higher levels of triglycerides in the bloodstream. These factors contribute to metabolic syndrome, a cluster of conditions that increase the risk of heart disease, diabetes, and stroke.

Unhealthy fats, including trans fats and saturated fats, are prevalent in fast food. Trans fats, in particular, are known to increase low-density lipoprotein (LDL) cholesterol levels while decreasing high-density lipoprotein (HDL) cholesterol levels. This imbalance accelerates the development of heart disease. Saturated fats, while less harmful than trans fats, still contribute to increased cholesterol levels and the risk of cardiovascular issues.

Long-Term Effects of Frequent Consumption

The cumulative effects of frequent fast-food consumption extend beyond immediate health risks. Over time, individuals who regularly consume fast food may experience significant weight gain, which can lead to obesity. Obesity itself is a risk factor for numerous chronic conditions, including joint problems, sleep apnea, and certain types of cancer.

Moreover, the dietary habits established through frequent fast-food consumption can have generational implications. Families that rely heavily on fast food may inadvertently influence their children's eating habits, perpetuating a cycle of poor nutrition and associated health risks. Children exposed to high-calorie, low-nutrient diets are more likely to develop obesity and related health issues at a younger age, setting the stage for lifelong struggles with chronic diseases.

Another long-term consequence is the strain on healthcare systems. The rising prevalence of chronic illnesses linked to poor dietary habits has increased the demand for medical interventions, ranging from medications to surgeries. This growing burden not only affects individual quality of life but also places significant financial and resource constraints on healthcare providers and society as a whole.

Mitigating the Risks

While the health risks associated with fast food are well-documented, they are not insurmountable. Awareness and education about the nutritional content of fast food can empower individuals to make informed choices. For instance, opting for smaller portion sizes, choosing menu items with fewer calories and less sodium, and supplementing fast food meals with fresh fruits and vegetables can help mitigate some of the negative effects.

Policy changes can also play a role in addressing the public health impact of fast food. Efforts to reduce the use of trans fats, limit the sodium content in processed foods, and improve food labeling practices have shown promise in promoting healthier eating habits. Additionally, public health campaigns that encourage cooking at home and increasing access to affordable, nutritious food options can help shift dietary patterns away from fast food dependency.

In conclusion, the chronic health issues linked to fast food consumption are a reflection of broader dietary and lifestyle trends. By understanding the connections between fast food and conditions such as diabetes, heart disease, and hypertension, individuals and communities can take proactive steps to reduce their risk and improve overall health. Addressing the excessive sodium, sugars, and unhealthy fats in fast food is essential to mitigating its long-term effects and fostering a healthier future.

Fast Food in America
"The Health Effects, Cultural Impacts, and Future of Convenience Eating"

Chapter 5

The Psychological Impact of Fast Food

- ☐ The addictive nature of fast food ingredients like sugar and fat.

- ☐ Emotional eating and the appeal of comfort foods.

- ☐ How marketing strategies tap into psychological triggers.

Fast food is more than just a convenient meal option; it has deeply ingrained psychological effects on consumers. From the addictive properties of its ingredients to its appeal as a source of comfort, fast food taps into human emotions and behaviors in powerful ways. This chapter explores the psychological impact of fast food by examining its addictive nature, the role it plays in emotional eating, and the marketing strategies that exploit psychological triggers to drive consumption.

The Addictive Nature of Fast-Food Ingredients

Fast food's widespread popularity can be partly attributed to the addictive qualities of its ingredients, such as sugar, fat, and salt. These elements are not merely flavor enhancers but chemical compounds that interact with the brain's reward system. When consumed, sugar triggers the release of dopamine, a neurotransmitter associated with pleasure and satisfaction. This reaction creates a sense of euphoria, encouraging repeated consumption to replicate the experience.

Fat, another key component in fast food, provides a rich texture and flavor profile that enhances palatability. Fat consumption

Fast Food in America
"The Health Effects, Cultural Impacts, and Future of Convenience Eating"

also activates the brain's reward system, making it difficult to resist high-fat foods. Similarly, salt amplifies flavors and creates a craving for more, contributing to the cycle of addiction. Together, these ingredients form a trifecta that is specifically engineered to be irresistible.

Scientists have noted that the combination of sugar, fat, and salt in fast food mirrors the effects of addictive substances, leading to behaviors similar to dependency. Over time, repeated exposure to these hyper-palatable foods can alter brain chemistry, making individuals more susceptible to cravings and overconsumption. This dependency is not only psychological but also physiological, as the body begins to expect and demand these foods.

Emotional Eating and the Appeal of Comfort Foods

Fast food is often associated with emotional eating, a behavior where individuals consume food as a way to cope with stress, sadness, or other emotional states. The convenience and accessibility of fast food make it an easy choice for those seeking comfort during challenging times. Moreover, the sensory experience of eating fast food—its flavors, textures, and even aromas—can provide a temporary sense of relief or happiness.

The concept of comfort foods is deeply rooted in psychology. These foods often evoke nostalgia or positive associations, such as childhood memories or celebrations. Fast food, with its consistent taste and branding, becomes a reliable source of comfort for many people. This emotional connection can lead to a pattern of using fast food as a coping mechanism, reinforcing its role in emotional eating.

Fast Food in America
"The Health Effects, Cultural Impacts, and Future of Convenience Eating"

Emotional eating, however, often leads to negative consequences. The temporary relief provided by fast food is usually followed by feelings of guilt or regret, particularly when it contributes to poor health or weight gain. This cycle can perpetuate a reliance on fast food, creating a feedback loop that is difficult to break.

Marketing Strategies and Psychological Triggers

The success of fast food is not only a result of its addictive ingredients but also the marketing strategies that tap into psychological triggers. Fast food companies invest heavily in advertising campaigns designed to appeal to emotions, desires, and subconscious needs.

One of the most effective strategies is the use of bright colors, such as red and yellow, in branding and packaging. These colors are known to stimulate appetite and evoke feelings of excitement and energy. Additionally, the use of jingles, slogans, and mascots creates a sense of familiarity and trust, making consumers more likely to choose fast food over other options.

Another key tactic is the promotion of value meals and limited time offers. These strategies create a sense of urgency and appeal to consumers' desire for a good deal, encouraging impulsive purchases. Fast food marketing also leverages social proof, showcasing crowded restaurants or celebrity endorsements to suggest that their products are highly desirable.

Marketing to children is another area where fast food companies excel. By incorporating toys, games, and characters into their advertising, they create a strong emotional bond with young consumers. This early exposure can influence lifelong eating habits, establishing a preference for fast food that persists into adulthood.

The Role of Social Media and Digital Marketing

In recent years, social media and digital platforms have become crucial tools for fast food marketing. These platforms allow for targeted advertising based on consumer behavior and preferences. By analyzing data, companies can tailor their messages to specific demographics, increasing the likelihood of engagement and purchase.

Social media campaigns often rely on user-generated content, such as photos or videos of fast-food items, to create a sense of community and belonging. Hashtags and challenges encourage consumers to share their experiences, effectively turning them into brand ambassadors. This type of marketing exploits the human need for social connection and validation, further solidifying fast food's place in daily life.

Long-Term Psychological Effects

The psychological impact of fast food extends beyond immediate gratification and emotional eating. Over time, habitual fast-food consumption can lead to changes in mindset and behavior. For example, the convenience of fast food may contribute to a preference for instant gratification, making it harder to adopt healthier eating habits that require planning and effort.

Additionally, the normalization of fast food in society can influence perceptions of what constitutes a "meal" or "normal eating." This shift in mindset can make it challenging for individuals to recognize the nutritional deficiencies or health risks associated with fast food. As a result, the long-term psychological effects of fast food are closely intertwined with its physical and societal impacts.

Conclusion

The psychological impact of fast food is a complex interplay of addiction, emotional eating, and strategic marketing. Its addictive ingredients, coupled with its role as a source of comfort, make it a compelling choice for many consumers. At the same time, marketing strategies exploit psychological triggers to drive consumption, creating habits that are difficult to break. Understanding these psychological dynamics is essential for addressing the broader implications of fast food on individual and societal well-being.

Fast Food in America
"The Health Effects, Cultural Impacts, and Future of Convenience Eating"

Chapter 6

Children, Fast Food, and Development

☐ The role of fast food in childhood nutrition and growth.

☐ Marketing strategies targeting children and their long-term effects.

☐ Connections between early fast food habits and adult health outcomes.

Fast food has become an integral part of many children's diets, significantly shaping their nutritional intake and overall health outcomes. As children are in critical stages of physical and mental development, the foods they consume play a crucial role in determining their growth trajectory and future well-being. Examining the interplay between fast food and childhood development reveals a complex web of nutritional, behavioral, and societal factors.

The Role of Fast Food in Childhood Nutrition and Growth

Childhood is a period of rapid growth, requiring adequate intake of essential nutrients such as vitamins, minerals, proteins, and healthy fats. Unfortunately, fast food often falls short in meeting these nutritional needs. Fast food meals are typically high in calories, unhealthy fats, sugars, and sodium while being low in fiber, vitamins, and other critical nutrients. This imbalance can lead to both immediate and long-term consequences for children's health.

Fast Food in America
"The Health Effects, Cultural Impacts, and Future of Convenience Eating"

The caloric density of fast food can contribute to excessive energy intake, often surpassing the daily caloric requirements for children. This overconsumption is exacerbated by the large portion sizes that have become a hallmark of fast-food culture. Simultaneously, the lack of nutrient diversity in such meals may lead to deficiencies in essential nutrients like calcium, iron, and vitamins A and D, which are vital for bone health, cognitive development, and immune function.

Moreover, regular consumption of fast food can displace healthier food choices. Children who frequently eat fast food may develop preferences for salty, sweet, and fatty flavors, potentially rejecting more nutritious options like fruits, vegetables, and whole grains. This dietary pattern not only affects their growth and development during childhood but also sets the stage for unhealthy eating habits in adulthood.

Marketing Strategies Targeting Children and Their Long-Term Effects

Fast food marketing has long recognized the value of children as a target demographic. Companies often employ strategies designed to capture children's attention and loyalty from an early age. Brightly colored packaging, playful mascots, and promotional toys are common features in marketing campaigns aimed at young consumers. These tactics create a strong association between fast food and fun, making the products highly appealing to children.

Television commercials, digital advertisements, and social media campaigns often emphasize the immediate gratification and enjoyment of fast food. Studies have shown that children exposed to fast food advertising are more likely to crave and request these foods, influencing their parents' purchasing decisions. This cycle not only increases immediate consumption but also establishes brand loyalty that can persist into adulthood.

The impact of such marketing extends beyond individual dietary choices. It contributes to a food environment where unhealthy options are normalized, making it harder for parents and caregivers to promote balanced eating habits. Additionally, the psychological appeal of fast-food marketing can exacerbate emotional eating behaviors, as children learn to associate food with comfort, reward, and celebration.

Connections Between Early Fast-Food Habits and Adult Health Outcomes

Early exposure to fast food can have lasting implications for health and well-being. Research indicates that dietary habits formed during childhood often carry over into adulthood. Children who consume fast food regularly are more likely to continue this pattern, increasing their risk of chronic health issues such as obesity, diabetes, and cardiovascular diseases.

One of the key concerns is the link between fast food consumption and childhood obesity. The high calorie and low nutrient density of fast-food meals contribute to weight gain, particularly when combined with sedentary lifestyles. Obesity during childhood is associated with a host of complications, including insulin resistance, high blood pressure, and joint problems, many of which persist into adulthood.

Beyond physical health, the long-term consequences of early fast-food consumption extend to mental and emotional well-being. Poor nutrition during critical developmental periods can impair cognitive function, academic performance, and emotional regulation. Moreover, the habit of turning to fast food for convenience or emotional comfort can create a cycle of unhealthy eating behaviors that are difficult to break.

Addressing these issues requires a multifaceted approach. Parents, educators, and policymakers play a vital role in shaping children's food environments and promoting healthier alternatives. Schools can implement nutrition education programs and provide balanced meal options, while community initiatives can increase access to fresh, affordable produce. On a broader scale, regulating marketing practices aimed at children could help reduce the pervasive influence of fast-food advertising.

The Importance of Parental Influence and Education

Parents and caregivers serve as the primary gatekeepers of children's diets, making their role critical in mitigating the impact of fast food. Modeling healthy eating behaviors and creating a home environment where nutritious foods are readily available can significantly influence children's food choices. For example, involving children in meal planning and preparation can make healthy eating more engaging and appealing.

Educating parents about the nutritional content of fast food and its potential health consequences is equally important. Many parents may underestimate the calorie and sodium content of fast-food meals or overestimate their nutritional value. Providing clear, accessible information about healthier alternatives can empower families to make informed decisions.

Community and Policy Interventions

Addressing the influence of fast food on childhood development requires systemic changes at the community and policy levels. Initiatives to improve access to healthy foods in underserved areas, such as urban food deserts, can help reduce reliance on fast food. Policies that regulate portion sizes, limit the marketing of unhealthy foods to children, and promote transparency in nutritional labeling can also make a significant impact.

Schools and childcare centers can serve as important venues for promoting healthy eating habits. Implementing guidelines for school lunches, limiting the availability of fast food on campus, and integrating nutrition education into the curriculum can help shape children's attitudes toward food and nutrition. Community programs that engage families in cooking classes, gardening projects, and other activities can further reinforce the importance of balanced diets.

Looking Ahead

The relationship between children and fast food is a complex issue with far-reaching implications for public health. While fast food offers convenience and affordability, its impact on childhood nutrition, growth, and development cannot be overlooked. By addressing the root causes of fast-food consumption and promoting healthier alternatives, society can help ensure that children have the foundation they need for a lifetime of health and well-being.

In conclusion, the intersection of fast food and childhood development highlights the need for a comprehensive approach that combines individual, familial, and societal efforts. Through education, policy change, and community support, it is possible to mitigate the negative effects of fast food and foster a healthier future for the next generation.

Fast Food in America
"The Health Effects, Cultural Impacts, and Future of Convenience Eating"

Chapter 7

Fast Food in Low-Income Communities

☐ The prevalence of fast food in economically disadvantaged areas.

☐ Barriers to accessing healthier food alternatives.

☐ How fast food impacts health equity and disparities.

Fast food has become a significant aspect of daily life in many economically disadvantaged areas, reflecting a complex interplay of accessibility, affordability, and cultural norms. The prevalence of fast-food establishments in these communities is not an accident but rather a result of economic and social dynamics that shape the availability of food choices. This chapter delves into the factors contributing to the dominance of fast food in low-income neighborhoods, the barriers residents face in accessing healthier options, and the broader implications for health equity and disparities.

The Prevalence of Fast Food in Economically Disadvantaged Areas

Low-income communities are often characterized by a high density of fast-food outlets. This phenomenon can be attributed to several factors. First, fast food chains strategically place their establishments in areas with high foot traffic and population density, often targeting neighborhoods where economic constraints make their low-cost offerings particularly appealing. The affordability and convenience of fast food create a dependable consumer base in these areas, ensuring steady revenue for the businesses.

Another contributing factor is the lack of full-service grocery stores or supermarkets, a phenomenon often referred to as "food deserts." These are areas where residents have limited access to affordable and nutritious food. Without nearby options for fresh fruits, vegetables, and whole grains, residents often turn to fast food as a primary source of meals. The proliferation of fast-food outlets in such areas exacerbates the problem, creating an environment where unhealthy eating habits are not just common but almost inevitable.

Barriers to Accessing Healthier Food Alternatives

Economic constraints are a primary barrier to accessing healthier food alternatives. Fresh produce and nutrient-dense foods are often more expensive than fast food items, making them inaccessible to individuals and families with limited budgets. Additionally, the time required to prepare healthy meals at home is a significant obstacle for those working multiple jobs or dealing with other time-intensive responsibilities.

Transportation is another critical barrier. In many low-income communities, residents may not have access to reliable transportation to reach supermarkets or farmers' markets located outside their immediate neighborhoods. This lack of mobility further restricts their food choices, making fast food establishments the most convenient option.

Educational disparities also play a role. Limited awareness or knowledge about nutrition and healthy eating can lead individuals to make choices that prioritize convenience over health. Marketing strategies by fast food companies often exploit

Fast Food in America
"The Health Effects, Cultural Impacts, and Future of Convenience Eating"

this lack of nutritional literacy, promoting their products as affordable, tasty, and satisfying without emphasizing the long-term health risks associated with frequent consumption.

How Fast Food Impacts Health Equity and Disparities

The dominance of fast food in low-income communities has profound implications for health equity. Chronic health conditions such as obesity, diabetes, and cardiovascular disease are disproportionately prevalent in these areas, driven in part by dietary patterns heavily reliant on fast food. These conditions not only affect individual health outcomes but also strain public health systems and widen existing health disparities.

Nutritional inequities contribute to a cycle of poverty and poor health. Individuals dealing with chronic illnesses may face increased medical expenses, reduced productivity, and limited job opportunities, further entrenching economic disadvantage. The intergenerational effects are also significant, as children raised in environments dominated by fast food are more likely to develop unhealthy eating habits and related health problems as they grow older.

Public health initiatives aimed at addressing these disparities often face challenges in implementation. Efforts to introduce healthier food options in low-income communities, such as subsidized grocery stores or community gardens, require substantial investment and community buy-in. However, when successfully implemented, these programs can play a crucial role in breaking the cycle of unhealthy eating and improving overall community health.

Fast Food in America
"The Health Effects, Cultural Impacts, and Future of Convenience Eating"

The Role of Policy and Advocacy

Addressing the prevalence of fast food in low-income communities requires a multifaceted approach that includes policy changes, community advocacy, and public education. Policy measures such as zoning laws to limit the density of fast-food outlets, subsidies for fresh food retailers, and taxation on unhealthy food products can create an environment that supports healthier choices.

Community advocacy is equally important. Grassroots organizations often play a vital role in raising awareness about nutritional issues and advocating for resources to improve food access. Educational campaigns that empower residents with knowledge about healthy eating and cooking can help shift dietary patterns and demand for better food options.

Finally, public-private partnerships can be instrumental in addressing food insecurity and promoting health equity. Collaborations between government agencies, non-profits, and private businesses can result in innovative solutions, such as mobile markets, meal programs, and urban agriculture initiatives, that bring fresh and affordable food to underserved areas.

A Path Forward

The relationship between fast food and low-income communities is a complex issue rooted in economic, social, and cultural factors. While the challenges are significant, they are not insurmountable. By addressing barriers to healthy eating and investing in solutions that promote food equity, it is possible to create environments where all individuals, regardless of income, have the opportunity to make nutritious choices.

Fast Food in America
"The Health Effects, Cultural Impacts, and Future of Convenience Eating"

Ultimately, the goal is to shift the narrative from one of limited options to one of empowerment and opportunity. By prioritizing health equity and supporting sustainable changes in food systems, society can work towards a future where fast food is not a necessity but a choice, and healthier alternatives are accessible to everyone.

Fast Food in America
"The Health Effects, Cultural Impacts, and Future of Convenience Eating"

Chapter 8

The Cultural and Social Influence of Fast Food

- ☐ How fast food reflects and shapes American cultural values.

- ☐ The social rituals and convenience associated with fast food dining.

- ☐ Fast food as a symbol of globalization and its role in American identity.

Fast food is not merely a type of cuisine; it is a cultural phenomenon that mirrors and molds societal norms and values. Its ubiquitous presence in American life has far-reaching implications, influencing everything from daily routines to national identity. Understanding how fast food reflects and shapes culture involves examining its role in social rituals, the values it embodies, and its broader influence on globalization.

Reflecting and Shaping American Cultural Values

Fast food has become a symbol of core American cultural values, including convenience, efficiency, and individualism. Rooted in the country's rapid pace of life, fast food epitomizes the desire for quick solutions to daily challenges. The industry's focus on speed and affordability aligns with a cultural emphasis on productivity and economic pragmatism.

Moreover, the rise of fast food reflects the societal embrace of standardization. With predictable menus and uniform service, fast food chains offer a sense of reliability in an otherwise

Fast Food in America
"The Health Effects, Cultural Impacts, and Future of Convenience Eating"

unpredictable world. This predictability fosters trust and comfort, particularly in a society where mobility and relocation are common.

The cultural emphasis on choice and personal freedom is also evident in fast food dining. Customers can customize meals, choose from diverse options, and decide where and when to eat. This flexibility caters to individual preferences and lifestyles, reinforcing the American ideal of self-determination.

Social Rituals and the Convenience of Fast-Food Dining

Fast food has embedded itself in the social fabric of American life. It serves as a backdrop for numerous social rituals, from family dinners to workplace lunches. Its affordability and accessibility make it an appealing choice for people from all walks of life.

For families, fast food offers a quick solution to the challenge of feeding everyone amidst busy schedules. It becomes a shared experience that fosters togetherness, even if only for a brief meal. For workers, fast food provides a convenient option for lunch breaks, allowing them to maximize productivity while satisfying hunger.

Fast food restaurants also serve as gathering spaces for communities. Whether hosting birthday parties or informal meetings, these venues facilitate social interaction. Their casual and approachable atmosphere makes them inclusive spaces where people can connect without formality.

The convenience of fast food extends beyond its speed and accessibility. Many fast-food establishments operate around the clock, accommodating the varied schedules of modern life. This

Fast Food in America
"The Health Effects, Cultural Impacts, and Future of Convenience Eating"

availability ensures that people can access food regardless of their circumstances, reinforcing its role as a practical choice.

Fast Food as a Symbol of Globalization

The influence of fast food transcends American borders, making it a global phenomenon. Its spread to other countries illustrates the cultural exportation of American values, including efficiency and consumer choice. Fast food establishments abroad often serve as symbols of modernity and economic progress, representing the appeal of American-style capitalism.

This globalization has created a two-way exchange of cultural influence. While fast food brings American practices to other nations, it also absorbs local flavors and customs, adapting menus to cater to regional tastes. This cultural hybridization demonstrates the industry's ability to integrate into diverse societies while maintaining its core identity.

However, the globalization of fast food has sparked debates about cultural homogenization. Critics argue that the proliferation of fast food erodes traditional culinary practices and diminishes cultural diversity. In contrast, supporters view it as a vehicle for cultural exchange, promoting cross-cultural understanding through food.

The Role of Fast Food in American Identity

Fast food has become a defining feature of American identity. Its origins and growth are intertwined with the nation's history, reflecting economic and social changes. From its early days as a response to urbanization and industrialization to its current status as a global force, fast food embodies the dynamic nature of American society.

Fast Food in America
"The Health Effects, Cultural Impacts, and Future of Convenience Eating"

The industry's marketing strategies have further solidified its cultural significance. Advertising campaigns often portray fast food as an integral part of the American experience, celebrating themes such as family, community, and patriotism. These narratives resonate with consumers, reinforcing the emotional connection between fast food and national identity.

Fast food's affordability and accessibility have also contributed to its cultural resonance. By providing a common dining experience for people across socioeconomic backgrounds, it fosters a sense of inclusivity and shared identity. This democratization of food reflects the American ideal of equality, even as disparities in access to healthier options persist.

Broader Cultural Impacts

The cultural influence of fast food extends beyond the dining table. It has inspired various aspects of popular culture, from films and television shows to music and art. These representations often highlight the industry's role in shaping societal norms, sometimes celebrating its convenience and other times critiquing its impact.

Fast food has also influenced broader lifestyle trends. The emphasis on speed and efficiency aligns with a fast-paced modern existence, shaping consumer expectations for other industries. For example, the concept of "fast" has extended to other services, such as fashion and technology, reflecting the pervasive influence of fast-food culture.

Moreover, fast food has played a role in shaping perceptions of health and wellness. Its prominence in discussions about nutrition and public health underscores its cultural significance. These debates often reflect broader societal values, such as

Fast Food in America
"The Health Effects, Cultural Impacts, and Future of Convenience Eating"

individual responsibility versus collective action, further illustrating the interconnectedness of fast food and culture.

Conclusion

Fast food's cultural and social influence is profound, shaping and reflecting the values of American society. From its role in daily routines to its global reach, it represents both the strengths and challenges of modern life. While it offers convenience and inclusivity, it also raises questions about health, sustainability, and cultural diversity. By understanding the cultural and social dimensions of fast food, we can better appreciate its impact on our lives and consider its implications for the future.

Fast Food in America
"The Health Effects, Cultural Impacts, and Future of Convenience Eating"

Chapter 9

Efforts to Address Health Concerns in Fast Food

- ☐ Industry responses to criticism, including healthier menu options.

- ☐ Public awareness campaigns and policy changes.

- ☐ The rise of fast-casual dining as a healthier alternative.

Fast food has long been associated with convenience and affordability, but it has also been criticized for its role in public health issues. Over time, the industry, policymakers, and consumers have made significant efforts to address these concerns. This chapter explores these initiatives, focusing on industry responses, public campaigns, and the emergence of fast-casual dining as a perceived healthier alternative.

Industry Responses to Criticism

One of the most significant responses from the fast-food industry to growing health concerns has been the introduction of healthier menu options. Recognizing the increasing demand for nutritious alternatives, many fast-food establishments began offering salads, grilled items, and reduced-calorie meals. While the core menu items often remain unchanged, these additions provide choices for health-conscious consumers.

Menu labeling has been another critical step. Nutritional information, such as calorie counts, is now displayed on menus and packaging in many establishments. This transparency allows consumers to make more informed decisions about their food choices. Studies have suggested that such labeling can influence purchasing behaviors, encouraging people to opt for lower-calorie options.

Reformulation of recipes has also been a focal point. Efforts to reduce sodium, trans fats, and added sugars in popular menu items have gained traction. These changes aim to improve the nutritional profile of fast food without significantly altering its taste, ensuring that it remains appealing to the target audience.

Public Awareness Campaigns

Public health organizations and advocacy groups have played a significant role in raising awareness about the health implications of fast-food consumption. Campaigns emphasizing the importance of balanced diets, portion control, and the risks associated with excessive consumption of processed foods have gained widespread attention.

Educational initiatives targeting schools and families aim to foster healthier eating habits from an early age. These programs often provide resources and tools to help individuals understand nutritional information and make healthier food choices. The focus on children is particularly important, as early dietary patterns can have lasting impacts on health.

The media has also been instrumental in shaping public perception of fast food. Documentaries, books, and articles highlighting the health risks associated with fast food have sparked widespread discussion. These narratives often emphasize the importance of moderation and the need for systemic change in food production and marketing practices.

Fast Food in America
"The Health Effects, Cultural Impacts, and Future of Convenience Eating"

Policy Changes and Regulation

Government policies and regulations have been pivotal in addressing health concerns related to fast food. Nutritional labeling requirements, bans on trans fats, and restrictions on marketing unhealthy foods to children are examples of regulatory measures implemented in various regions.

Taxes on sugary drinks and other unhealthy food items have been introduced in some areas as a deterrent. These taxes aim to reduce consumption while generating revenue for public health initiatives. While controversial, such measures have shown promise in curbing unhealthy eating habits.

School nutrition programs have also undergone significant reforms. Policies promoting the inclusion of fruits, vegetables, and whole grains in school meals, while limiting the availability of high-calorie, low-nutrient foods, reflect a broader commitment to improving childhood nutrition.

The Rise of Fast-Casual Dining

The emergence of fast-casual dining establishments has been one of the most notable trends in the food industry. Positioned between traditional fast food and full-service restaurants, fast-casual dining offers a balance of convenience, quality, and perceived health benefits.

Fast-casual menus often feature fresh ingredients, customizable options, and a focus on transparency. These establishments typically emphasize the sourcing of ingredients, highlighting terms like "organic," "locally sourced," and "non-GMO." This approach appeals to consumers seeking healthier and more sustainable dining options.

Fast Food in America
"The Health Effects, Cultural Impacts, and Future of Convenience Eating"

Portion control and variety are other hallmarks of fast-casual dining. Many of these establishments allow customers to tailor their meals to suit their dietary preferences and needs, making it easier to adhere to specific nutritional goals.

Challenges and Critiques

Despite these efforts, challenges remain in addressing health concerns related to fast food. Critics argue that healthier menu options and nutritional labeling are not enough to counteract the pervasive influence of fast-food culture. The affordability and accessibility of traditional fast-food items often outweigh the appeal of healthier alternatives, particularly in low-income communities.

There is also skepticism about the authenticity of industry-led initiatives. Some view these efforts as superficial, designed more to enhance public relations than to effect meaningful change. For instance, while some fast-food establishments promote healthier items, these options often constitute a small fraction of overall sales.

Moreover, public health campaigns and policy measures face resistance from various stakeholders. The food industry's economic influence, coupled with differing opinions on the role of government regulation, complicates efforts to implement and sustain meaningful change.

The Role of Technology and Innovation

Technology has played a significant role in advancing efforts to address health concerns in fast food. Mobile apps and online platforms providing nutritional information, meal customization, and dietary tracking have empowered consumers to make more informed choices.

Fast Food in America
"The Health Effects, Cultural Impacts, and Future of Convenience Eating"

Innovations in food technology have also contributed to the development of healthier fast-food options. Plant-based proteins, alternative cooking methods, and advancements in food preservation techniques are reshaping the nutritional landscape of fast food. These developments reflect a growing demand for healthier and more sustainable food options.

Future Directions

Looking ahead, the fast-food industry is likely to continue evolving in response to health concerns and consumer demands. Greater emphasis on plant-based and environmentally friendly options, coupled with advancements in nutritional science, could lead to a more health-conscious fast-food culture.

Collaboration between industry, policymakers, and public health organizations will be crucial in driving progress. By addressing systemic barriers and fostering a culture of health and wellness, it is possible to mitigate the negative health impacts associated with fast food while preserving its benefits of convenience and affordability.

In conclusion, efforts to address health concerns in fast food reflect a complex interplay of industry initiatives, public awareness, and regulatory measures. While significant progress has been made, ongoing challenges underscore the need for continued innovation, collaboration, and commitment to public health.

Fast Food in America
"The Health Effects, Cultural Impacts, and Future of Convenience Eating"

Chapter 10

The Role of Technology in the Future of Fast Food

- [ ] The influence of apps, delivery services, and automation on consumption.

- [ ] How technology could improve nutritional transparency and customization.

- [ ] Innovations aimed at making fast food healthier and more sustainable.

In recent decades, technology has significantly reshaped industries worldwide, and fast food is no exception. From the way food is prepared and delivered to the methods by which consumers interact with brands, technology is revolutionizing every aspect of the fast-food experience. This chapter explores the impact of technological innovations on fast food, focusing on their influence on consumption patterns, improvements in nutritional transparency and customization, and the potential for creating healthier and more sustainable options.

The Rise of Apps and Delivery Services

One of the most prominent technological shifts in the fast-food industry is the proliferation of mobile applications and online delivery services. These tools provide unparalleled convenience, allowing consumers to order meals with just a few taps on their smartphones. The ease of access has expanded the reach of fast food, enabling brands to serve customers beyond the confines of physical locations. This expansion has increased consumption rates, particularly among urban populations seeking quick and convenient meal options.

The integration of delivery platforms into the fast-food ecosystem has also changed the dynamics of food service. These platforms offer features such as real-time tracking, customizable menus, and loyalty programs, further incentivizing frequent use. However, this convenience comes with implications for health, as the accessibility of calorie-dense meals may encourage overconsumption. At the same time, the availability of nutritional information on apps provides an opportunity for consumers to make more informed choices, which can mitigate some of these concerns.

Automation in Food Preparation and Service

Automation is another transformative force in the fast-food industry. Automated systems are being introduced at various stages of the food preparation and service process, from robotic kitchen equipment to self-order kiosks. These technologies improve efficiency, reduce wait times, and minimize human error, leading to a more consistent product. Automation also allows for greater precision in portion control, which can have implications for calorie management and cost efficiency.

Self-order kiosks, for example, offer a personalized ordering experience, enabling customers to modify their meals to suit dietary preferences or restrictions. This level of customization is particularly appealing in an era where consumers increasingly demand transparency and control over their food choices. Additionally, automated systems can collect valuable data on consumer preferences, allowing businesses to refine their offerings and better meet customer demands.

Fast Food in America
"The Health Effects, Cultural Impacts, and Future of Convenience Eating"

Enhancing Nutritional Transparency and Customization

As consumers become more health-conscious, the demand for nutritional transparency has grown. Technology plays a vital role in addressing this need by providing detailed nutritional information through digital platforms. Mobile apps and in-store kiosks often display calorie counts, ingredient lists, and allergen warnings, empowering consumers to make informed decisions about their meals.

Customization is another area where technology is making strides. Interactive menus allow customers to tailor their orders by adjusting portion sizes, substituting ingredients, or selecting healthier preparation methods. For instance, customers might opt for grilled rather than fried options or choose smaller portion sizes to reduce calorie intake. These innovations not only enhance the dining experience but also promote healthier eating habits.

Innovations for Healthier Fast Food

Technological advancements are paving the way for healthier fast-food options. One significant trend is the development of alternative ingredients, such as plant-based proteins and low-calorie sweeteners. These innovations enable fast-food providers to offer menu items that cater to diverse dietary needs without compromising on taste or quality.

Additionally, technology is driving improvements in food processing techniques, resulting in products that retain more nutrients while reducing harmful components like trans fats and excessive sodium. For example, advanced cooking methods such as air frying and sous-vide are being explored to create healthier meal options without sacrificing flavor or texture.

Fast Food in America
"The Health Effects, Cultural Impacts, and Future of Convenience Eating"

The Push for Sustainability

Sustainability is becoming a critical concern for the fast-food industry, and technology is playing a crucial role in addressing environmental challenges. Innovations in packaging, for instance, are reducing waste and promoting the use of biodegradable materials. Smart inventory management systems are helping businesses minimize food waste by accurately forecasting demand and optimizing supply chains.

Furthermore, advances in agricultural technology, such as vertical farming and precision agriculture, are enabling more sustainable sourcing of ingredients. These methods reduce the environmental footprint of food production and ensure a consistent supply of fresh, high-quality ingredients. The adoption of renewable energy solutions in fast-food operations is another step toward achieving greater sustainability.

The Future of Fast-Food Dining

Looking ahead, the integration of emerging technologies promises to further transform the fast-food industry. Artificial intelligence (AI) and machine learning are being utilized to predict consumer preferences, streamline operations, and enhance customer engagement. Virtual and augmented reality technologies may also play a role in creating immersive dining experiences, blurring the lines between physical and digital spaces.

Blockchain technology is another innovation with potential applications in fast food. By providing a transparent and secure record of supply chain activities, blockchain can enhance food safety, ensure ethical sourcing, and build consumer trust. This

Fast Food in America
"The Health Effects, Cultural Impacts, and Future of Convenience Eating"

level of accountability aligns with the growing demand for socially responsible and environmentally friendly practices.

Balancing Innovation with Responsibility

While technology offers numerous benefits, it also presents challenges that must be addressed to ensure its responsible use. For instance, the increased reliance on delivery services and packaging materials raises concerns about environmental sustainability. Similarly, the accessibility of fast food through digital platforms could exacerbate health issues if not accompanied by effective public education and policy measures.

The fast-food industry has a unique opportunity to leverage technology to promote healthier and more sustainable eating habits. By prioritizing innovation that aligns with consumer needs and societal goals, businesses can create a future where convenience and well-being coexist.

Conclusion

Technology is reshaping the fast-food landscape, influencing how food is prepared, delivered, and consumed. From enhancing nutritional transparency to driving sustainability, technological advancements are unlocking new possibilities for the industry. As these innovations continue to evolve, the challenge lies in balancing convenience and efficiency with the need for healthier and more responsible practices. The future of fast food will be defined not only by its ability to adapt to changing consumer demands but also by its commitment to creating a positive impact on health, culture, and the environment.

Fast Food in America
"The Health Effects, Cultural Impacts, and Future of Convenience Eating"

Chapter 11

Environmental Consequences of Fast Food

☐ The ecological impact of fast food production and packaging.

☐ Issues with waste management, deforestation, and emissions.

☐ Emerging trends in sustainable practices and eco-friendly solutions..

Fast food, a ubiquitous part of modern dining culture, has significant implications for the environment. The production, distribution, and consumption of fast food contribute to a wide range of ecological challenges, from resource depletion to pollution and waste management issues. As the industry continues to evolve, so does its environmental footprint, making this a critical area of examination and innovation.

The Ecological Impact of Fast-Food Production and Packaging

Fast food production requires extensive natural resources, including land, water, and energy. The industrial-scale farming of livestock and crops used in fast food products is one of the leading contributors to deforestation and habitat loss. Vast tracts of land are cleared to grow feed crops like corn and soybeans or to provide grazing areas for livestock. This deforestation not only reduces biodiversity but also releases significant amounts of carbon dioxide into the atmosphere, exacerbating climate change.

Fast Food in America
"The Health Effects, Cultural Impacts, and Future of Convenience Eating"

Moreover, the high demand for meat in fast food has a ripple effect on water usage. Raising livestock is water-intensive, with thousands of gallons required to produce a single pound of beef. Similarly, processing plants consume large quantities of water, further straining local water supplies. Energy use is another concern, as the transportation of ingredients and operation of production facilities rely heavily on fossil fuels.

Packaging adds another layer of environmental impact. The widespread use of single-use plastics, paper products, and Styrofoam in fast food contributes to waste accumulation in landfills and oceans. These materials often take centuries to decompose, and improper disposal leads to microplastic pollution, which affects marine ecosystems and enters the food chain.

Issues with Waste Management, Deforestation, and Emissions

The fast-food industry generates substantial waste, much of which ends up in landfills or as litter. The reliance on disposable packaging and utensils creates a steady stream of trash that cities and municipalities struggle to manage. Recycling rates for fast food packaging remain low due to contamination from food residues and the complexity of recycling mixed materials.

Deforestation linked to fast food production has far-reaching consequences. The clearing of forests for agricultural expansion disrupts carbon storage systems, releasing greenhouse gases that contribute to global warming. Additionally, it disrupts local weather patterns and water cycles, affecting nearby communities and ecosystems.

Fast Food in America
"The Health Effects, Cultural Impacts, and Future of Convenience Eating"

Emissions from fast food production are another significant concern. Livestock farming produces large amounts of methane, a potent greenhouse gas. Transportation and processing add further emissions, creating a complex web of environmental challenges. These emissions not only drive climate change but also affect air quality, posing health risks to nearby populations.

Emerging Trends in Sustainable Practices and Eco-Friendly Solutions

In response to growing environmental concerns, the fast-food industry has begun exploring more sustainable practices. Plant-based alternatives to traditional meat products are gaining popularity, offering a lower-impact option for consumers. These alternatives require fewer resources to produce and generate fewer greenhouse gas emissions compared to conventional meat.

Efforts to reduce packaging waste are also underway. Biodegradable and compostable packaging materials are being developed to replace traditional plastics and Styrofoam. Some establishments are adopting reusable packaging systems or incentivizing customers to bring their own containers, helping to reduce the overall waste stream.

Innovations in waste management are addressing the challenges of food and packaging disposal. Composting programs for organic waste and advanced recycling technologies for mixed materials are being implemented in some regions. These initiatives aim to divert waste from landfills and promote a circular economy.

Sustainable sourcing is another area of focus. Ethical and environmentally friendly farming practices, such as regenerative

Fast Food in America
"The Health Effects, Cultural Impacts, and Future of Convenience Eating"

agriculture, are being encouraged to mitigate the environmental impact of food production. These practices emphasize soil health, water conservation, and reduced chemical use, benefiting both the environment and the farmers involved.

The Role of Consumer Awareness and Policy Changes

Consumer awareness plays a vital role in driving change within the fast-food industry. As more people become informed about the environmental consequences of their food choices, demand for sustainable options increases. Educational campaigns and transparent labeling can empower consumers to make choices that align with their values, encouraging the industry to adopt greener practices.

Policy changes are also instrumental in addressing the environmental impact of fast food. Governments and regulatory bodies can implement measures such as carbon taxes, waste reduction mandates, and incentives for sustainable practices. These policies create a framework for accountability and innovation, ensuring that environmental concerns are prioritized.

Balancing Convenience and Responsibility

The fast-food industry faces the challenge of balancing the convenience it offers with the responsibility to minimize its environmental footprint. While convenience remains a driving factor for consumers, many are willing to support brands that demonstrate a commitment to sustainability. By integrating eco-friendly practices into their operations, fast food establishments can meet this demand while contributing to broader environmental goals.

Fast Food in America
"The Health Effects, Cultural Impacts, and Future of Convenience Eating"

Conclusion

The environmental consequences of fast food are profound and multifaceted, spanning issues of resource consumption, waste generation, and emissions. However, the growing awareness and adoption of sustainable practices signal a shift towards a more eco-conscious future. By addressing these challenges through innovation, policy changes, and consumer engagement, the fast-food industry can play a pivotal role in promoting environmental stewardship and sustainability.

Fast Food in America
"The Health Effects, Cultural Impacts, and Future of Convenience Eating"

Chapter 12

The Future of Fast Food and Health

- ☐ Predictions for how fast food will evolve to meet health conscious demands.

- ☐ The potential role of plant-based and lab-grown alternatives.

- ☐ How societal attitudes toward fast food might change in the coming decades

As societal priorities shift toward healthier lifestyles and environmental sustainability, the fast-food industry is likely to undergo significant transformations. These changes will be driven by consumer demand, technological innovation, and a growing awareness of the health and environmental implications of dietary choices. While fast food has traditionally been associated with convenience and indulgence, its future may hold a balance between these qualities and a commitment to health and sustainability.

Evolving to Meet Health-Conscious Demands

The increasing prevalence of health-conscious consumers is shaping the trajectory of the fast-food industry. Rising awareness of the links between diet and chronic health conditions such as obesity, diabetes, and heart disease has prompted individuals to seek out healthier dining options. In response, the industry is likely to prioritize nutritional transparency and offer more health-focused menu items.

Fast Food in America
"The Health Effects, Cultural Impacts, and Future of Convenience Eating"

One potential trend is the incorporation of nutrient-dense, minimally processed ingredients. Fast food establishments may shift toward using whole grains, lean proteins, and fresh produce to appeal to health-conscious customers. Additionally, there could be a greater emphasis on portion control and calorie-conscious meals. The availability of customizable options, such as allowing consumers to select ingredients tailored to their dietary needs, is another likely development.

Plant-Based and Lab-Grown Alternatives

The demand for plant-based and lab-grown foods is gaining momentum, reflecting broader trends toward sustainability and animal welfare. Plant-based proteins, derived from ingredients such as legumes, grains, and vegetables, are expected to become a staple in fast food offerings. These alternatives mimic the taste and texture of traditional meat products while offering a more environmentally friendly footprint.

Lab-grown meat, produced through cellular agriculture, represents another groundbreaking innovation. This technology allows for the creation of real meat products without the environmental and ethical concerns associated with traditional animal farming. Although still in its early stages, lab-grown meat has the potential to revolutionize the fast-food industry by providing consumers with guilt-free indulgence.

Fast Food in America
"The Health Effects, Cultural Impacts, and Future of Convenience Eating"

The rise of these alternatives may also encourage the industry to experiment with hybrid products, combining plant-based and lab-grown components to create novel and appealing menu items. These innovations could address the dual demand for sustainability and health, positioning fast food establishments as leaders in the evolving food landscape.

Societal Attitudes Toward Fast Food

As health awareness continues to grow, societal attitudes toward fast food are likely to evolve. Historically viewed as a convenient but unhealthy choice, fast food may increasingly be associated with innovation and adaptability. This shift will depend on the industry's ability to align itself with emerging values, such as wellness, ethical consumption, and environmental stewardship.

Educational initiatives may play a crucial role in changing perceptions. By providing consumers with clear and accurate information about the nutritional content of their offerings, fast food establishments can foster trust and promote informed decision-making. Partnerships with health organizations or participation in public health campaigns could further enhance the industry's reputation.

Moreover, as younger generations prioritize ethical and sustainable practices, they may influence the fast-food market by demanding accountability from brands. These demands could lead to widespread adoption of environmentally friendly packaging, waste reduction strategies, and responsible sourcing of ingredients.

The Role of Technology

Technological advancements will likely be pivotal in shaping the future of fast food and health. Digital platforms and apps can enable greater customization and convenience, allowing consumers to tailor meals to their nutritional preferences. Artificial intelligence may also play a role in streamlining operations and personalizing marketing efforts.

Emerging technologies in food science, such as precision fermentation and 3D food printing, could introduce entirely new possibilities for fast food. These innovations may result in the development of nutrient-enhanced products designed to support specific health goals, such as boosting immunity or improving gut health.

Global Influences and Cross-Cultural Trends

The globalization of fast food has already led to the blending of culinary traditions, and this trend is expected to continue. As consumers seek diverse and flavorful options, fast food menus may incorporate a wider range of international cuisines. These offerings can be adapted to meet health-conscious demands, introducing nutrient-rich ingredients and traditional preparation methods.

Cross-cultural influences may also inspire innovations in meal composition, such as smaller portion sizes or the inclusion of side dishes that emphasize balance and variety. By drawing on global culinary traditions, the fast-food industry can offer options that are both healthful and culturally resonant.

Challenges and Opportunities

Despite these promising developments, the fast food industry faces challenges in balancing profitability with health and sustainability. Transitioning to healthier ingredients and sustainable practices may involve higher production costs, which could impact affordability. Addressing these challenges will require creative solutions, such as leveraging economies of scale or investing in cost-effective technologies.

Public policies and regulations may also influence the industry's trajectory. Governments and health organizations may implement measures to encourage healthier eating, such as imposing taxes on unhealthy products or offering incentives for nutritious alternatives. Collaboration between the industry and policymakers could lead to initiatives that benefit both businesses and consumers.

Conclusion

The future of fast food lies at the intersection of health, technology, and sustainability. As consumer priorities shift and innovations emerge, the industry has the opportunity to redefine itself as a force for positive change. By embracing these trends and addressing the challenges

Fast Food in America
"The Health Effects, Cultural Impacts, and Future of Convenience Eating"

ahead, fast food can continue to provide the convenience and enjoyment it is known for while contributing to a healthier and more sustainable world. This transformation will not only reshape the industry but also influence broader societal attitudes toward food and health in the years to come.

Fast Food in America
"The Health Effects, Cultural Impacts, and Future of Convenience Eating"

Final Thoughts

Fast food has undeniably become a defining element of American culture, blending convenience, affordability, and mass appeal. Its evolution mirrors the rapid pace of industrialization, urbanization, and technological advancements that have shaped modern society. What began as a solution to meet the demands of a fast-paced lifestyle has transformed into a global phenomenon, influencing dietary habits, cultural values, and economic systems.

The health effects of fast food have been a topic of intense scrutiny. High levels of sodium, unhealthy fats, and sugars commonly found in these meals contribute to chronic health issues such as obesity, diabetes, and heart disease. While these concerns have raised public awareness, they also serve as a reminder of the importance of informed choices and balanced nutrition. The cultural impact of fast food, however, extends far beyond its nutritional profile. It has redefined the way Americans view mealtime, replacing traditional, home-cooked meals with quick, on-the-go options that reflect the modern desire for efficiency and convenience.

Fast food's role in society is complex, touching on issues of health equity, environmental sustainability, and psychological well-being. In low-income communities, the prevalence of fast food underscores the broader challenges of access to affordable, nutritious food. At the same time, the environmental consequences of fast food—ranging from agricultural practices to waste management—highlight the need for systemic change. As the industry continues to adapt to these challenges, the rise of plant-based and sustainable options signals a shift toward a more conscientious approach to fast food consumption.

Fast Food in America
"The Health Effects, Cultural Impacts, and Future of Convenience Eating"

Looking forward, the future of fast food will likely reflect broader societal shifts. Health-conscious consumers, technological innovations, and environmental considerations are already shaping the industry's trajectory. Advances in food science, such as lab-grown meat and eco-friendly packaging, offer promising alternatives to traditional practices. Furthermore, the increasing demand for transparency and accountability may redefine the relationship between consumers and the fast-food industry.

Fast food is more than a meal—it is a reflection of societal values, challenges, and aspirations. By understanding its history, examining its impacts, and envisioning its future, we can better navigate the choices we make in our daily lives. Ultimately, the story of fast food in America is not just about what we eat, but about who we are and who we strive to become.

Fast Food in America
"The Health Effects, Cultural Impacts, and Future of Convenience Eating"

Notes

Fast Food in America
"The Health Effects, Cultural Impacts, and Future of Convenience Eating"

Notes

Fast Food in America
"The Health Effects, Cultural Impacts, and Future of Convenience Eating"

Notes

____

____

____

____

____

____

____

____

____

____

Fast Food in America
"The Health Effects, Cultural Impacts, and Future of Convenience Eating"

Notes

Fast Food in America
"The Health Effects, Cultural Impacts, and Future of Convenience Eating"

Notes

Fast Food in America
"The Health Effects, Cultural Impacts, and Future of Convenience Eating"

Notes

Notes

Fast Food in America
"The Health Effects, Cultural Impacts, and Future of Convenience Eating"

Notes